The Met Flex Dietary habits:Burn More Calories and Better Fuel.

by

Mark T.Riggs

Table of contents

Introduction

The Met Flex eating plan places a strong emphasis on metabolic inflexibility, or the capability to snappily switch between burning fats and carbohydrates for energy. By encouraging the body's ingrain capacity to acclimate to colorful energy sources, this strategy supports health and weight operation. Met Flex diets frequently emphasize whole foods, limit refined carbohydrates and sweets, and include moderate quantities of healthy fats and protein. In order to ameliorate metabolic inflexibility, it may also number intermittent fasting or time- confined feeding. Before making any big salutary changes, it's generally a good idea to speak with a medical guru or certified dietician. Then are some pointers that encourage metabolic rigidity.

1. Consume a healthy diet Include a range of entire foods similar as complex carbohydrates, spare proteins, healthy fats, and complex carbohydrates, too. This makes it possible to guarantee that your body gets all the nutrients it requires to operate at its stylish.

2. Engage in intermittent fasting, a diet strategy that alternates between times of eating and dieting. By tutoring your body to effectively burn stored fat for energy during fasting ages, it can help enhance metabolic inflexibility. Include HIIT(high-intensity interval training) Your metabolism will be boosted and your body will burn further fat if you include HIIT exercises in your fitness authority.

3.It encourages metabolic inflexibility by mixing brief bursts of vigorous exercise with rest ages.

4. Avoid spending too important time sitting down because it can harm your metabolism. Include regular breaks for movement during the day, similar as standing up, stretching, or taking a quick perambulation.

5. Stay doused It's pivotal to get enough water to keep an effective metabolism. It facilitates nutrient immersion, energy product, and digestion.

1: What Is Metabolic Flexibility?

Metabolic adaptability is the capacity to answer or adjust to restrictive changes in metabolic interest. This wide idea has been proliferated to make sense of insulin opposition and components overseeing fuel choice among glucose and unsaturated fats, featuring the metabolic resoluteness of corpulence and type 2 diabetes. In equal, contemporary activity physiology research has assisted with recognizing potential systems fundamental modified fuel digestion in weight and diabetes. Propels in 'omics' advances have additionally animated extra fundamental and clinical-translational exploration to additionally grill systems for worked on metabolic adaptability in skeletal muscle and fat tissue with the objective to forestall and treat metabolic illnesses.

Metabolic adaptability depicts the capacity of a creature to answer or adjust as per changes in metabolic or energy interest as well as the predominant circumstances or action. It was first utilized as a term portraying the expanded limit of helminthes, a parasitic worm, to produce substance energy and key metabolites either vigorously or by utilizing anaerobic breaths to give it more prominent adaptability and metabolic adaptability to answer and adjust to natural changes in its living space.

A metabolically adaptable state exists when there is a quick switch among glucose and unsaturated fats during the progress between the fed and fasting state. This adaptability in fuel decision effectively forestalls hyperglycemia following a feast and at the same time guarantees a sufficient measure of blood glucose is accessible for conveyance to the mind and only glycolytic tissues during fasting. The cutting edge period is portrayed by persistent overnutrition in which a combination of powers is conveyed to the mitochondria in an unabated way in this manner uncoupling the dining experience and starvation circumstance. The consistent deluge of fuel prompts amassing of lessening reciprocals in the mitochondria and an expansion in the mitochondrial layer potential. These progressions make a microenvironment encouraging the age of receptive oxygen species and different metabolites prompting injurious protein change, cell injury, and eventually clinical sickness. Insulin opposition may likewise assume an essential part in this harmful impact. The irregularity between mitochondrial energy conveyance and use is exacerbated with an inactive way of life. Moves that reestablish energy balance across the mitochondria actuate pathways that eliminate or fix harmed particles and reestablish the pliancy normal for typical energy digestion. Promptly accessible systems to keep up with energy balance across the mitochondria incorporate activity, different types of caloric limitation, organization of sodium-glucose cotransporter-2 inhibitors, cold openness, and hypobaric hypoxia.

The post-absorptive state is described by a diminishing in insulin levels and expanded glucagon emission in light of decreases in plasma glucose. Glucagon animates glycogenolysis causing arrival of glucose while decreases in insulin decline transport of glucose into skeletal muscle and adipocytes; accordingly guaranteeing satisfactory measures of blood glucose accessibility for conveyance to the cerebrum and solely glycolytic tissues like erythrocytes, the kidney medulla, bone marrow, and fringe nerves.Liver glucose-6-phosphatase eliminates the phosphate bunch from glucose 6-phosphate producing free glucose, which is delivered straightforwardly into the bloodstream.Because skeletal muscle needs glucose-6-phosphatase, muscle glycogen should initially be processed to lactate, which is delivered into the flow and resynthesized into glucose by the liver and kidney. Diminished insulin levels likewise enact lipolysis making unsaturated fats accessible to act as an elective fuel for skeletal muscle. Oxidation of unsaturated fats creates acetyl CoA and nicotinamide adenine dinucleotide (NADH), which allosterically and through actuation of pyruvate dehydrogenase kinase hinders the synergist movement of the pyruvate dehydrogenase complex, in this way guaranteeing that the little amount of skeletal muscle glucose take-up isn't totally oxidized by means of the citrus extract cycle however is specially used to pyruvate and lactate and changed back over completely to glucose in the liver.Decreased section of acetyl CoA into the citrus extract cycle restricts the stockpile of citrate accessible for send out from the mitochondria to the cytoplasm, consequently bringing down the degrees of malonyl CoA. Accordingly, unsaturated fat oxidation is animated through expanded carnitine palmitoyltransferase I movement, which controls the passage and oxidation of long chain unsaturated fats in the mitochondria. The shift to unsaturated fat assembly and oxidation in the liver gives energy to fuel glucose creation by means of the Cori cycle. The early dependence on Cori cycle action in the post-absorptive state saves protein by saving the requirement for amino corrosive antecedents for gluconeogenesis. As the span of the post-absorptive state extends, muscle proteolysis is expected to supply amino acids for liver gluconeogenesis. Hence, a liberal stockpile of glucose in the fed state prompts expanded glycolysis, glucose take-up and capacity, and concealment of unsaturated fat oxidation, while unsaturated fat oxidation is the favored wellspring of fuel during fasting, saving glucose for use by the mind. Metabolic intermediates emerging from glucose oxidation are negative controllers of fat catabolism as well as the other way around. Special utilization of carb or lipid as fuel and exchanging between the two probably developed from conditions where supported times of energy shortage went before the absorptive state. Free correspondence and cooperativity between the contending fuel sources guarantees that energy organic market are adjusted at the level of the mitochondria. As of now, the apportioning of various energy sources is not generally isolated because of persistent overnutrition without mediating times of diminished food consumption. Unremitting conveyance of glucose all the while alongside unsaturated fats makes an unbendable state in the mitochondria in which electrons are coercively fed into the respiratory chain eventuating in mitochondrial and cell injury.This harmful impact is amplified when joined by less energy interest (dormancy). At the point when energy supply surpasses energy interest across the mitochondria, an unbending and blocked state is made inclining toward negative wellbeing results. Insulin opposition may likewise assume an essential part in making this irregularity.

Impeded Fuel Exchanging With Persistent Overnutrition
Changes in fuel inclination as one advances among taking care of and fasting can be identified by changes in the respiratory remainder. This component reflects cell paces of CO_2 creation comparative with O_2consumption diminishing toward 0.7 with more noteworthy measures of unsaturated fat digestion and expanding to more prominent than 1 when carb digestion is prevailing. Utilization of a feast enhanced with

carbs evokes a flood in the respiratory remainder mirroring the transcendence of glucose oxidation while the remainder falls in the post-absorptive period mirroring a shift to unsaturated fat oxidation. Thoughtfully, the size of the motions are more articulated in a metabolically solid individual mirroring the capacity to unreservedly switch between the oxidative fuels.2,10,11 With overnutrition, the motions are dulled, as there is determined oxidation of a combination of carbon powers.

Backhanded calorimetry studies analyzing the equilibrium between glucose and unsaturated fat take-up across the leg show aggravations in skeletal muscle fuel elements in stout subjects when contrasted and solid controls. Utilizing a hyperinsulinemic euglycemic clasp to mirror the fed state, glucose take-up in solid subjects increments 10-crease with commitments from both capacity and oxidation, though unsaturated fat take-up decisively diminishes, which is reflected by an expansion in the respiratory remainder (RQ) from roughly 0.8 to 1.0. Conversely, glucose take-up is dulled in stout subjects during the clasp. The pace of fat oxidation in skeletal muscle of large people is lower during fasting. The gauge RQ of 0.9 in large subjects neglects to change in light of the cinch recommending a rigid state where a combination of fats and carbs keep on being oxidized notwithstanding the changing nourishing setting. A restriction of these examinations is that they were led under cinched conditions as opposed to overabundance supplement consuumption. Furthermore, inordinate nourishment changes metabolic adaptability, which might be both a reason and outcome of infection.

Concentrates on in both creature models and people recommend taking care of a high-fat eating routine causes a versatile expansion in β-oxidation without an equal expansion in compounds of the carboxyl corrosive (TCA) cycle. This distinction results in mitochondrial amassing of not completely oxidized lipid species reflected by quantifiable expansions in acylcarnitines. Collection of these and other deficiently oxidized substrates cause mitochondrial stress and at last might prompt insulin obstruction. Notwithstanding, in the event that the high-fat eating regimen is joined by expanded energy interest, aggregation of deficiently processed substrates is limited and insulin responsiveness is standardized

Firmness being used of substrates causes aggravations in branch chain amino corrosive (BCAA) (leucine, isoleucine, and valine) homeostasis portrayed in conditions of constant overnutrition. Not at all like other amino acids which are widely used in the liver following gastrointestinal assimilation, low degrees of hepatic mitochondrial expanded chain aminotransferase permits these amino acids to be conveyed into the foundational flow where they are first utilized in quite a while. Expanded degrees of BCAA assume a contributory part being developed of insulin opposition in fat people. Decreases in adipocyte digestion prompts expanded circling levels of BCAA. In the setting of overnutrition, glucose and unsaturated fat take-up by adipocytes might be the general reason for downregulated BCAA catabolic catalysts. Weakened brown fat tissue action adds to raised levels in a stout or diabetic state. The extended pool of BCAA is moved to the liver and, specifically, skeletal muscle as the essential site for digestion. in these tissues creates propionyl CoA and succinyl CoA, which can fill the citrus extract cycle through the course of anaplerosis. This impact adds to wasteful oxidation of unsaturated fats causing gathering of deficiently oxidized metabolites of unsaturated fats and BCAA, especially in the setting of high-fat eating regimen. Glucose use in muscle is pointless in the setting of supplement overabundance prompting diminished glucose oxidation and at last glucose narrow mindedness. Also, gathering of BCAA metabolites can constitutively enact mammalian objective of rapamycin (mTOR) causing determined insulin receptor substrate 1 phosphorylation by mammalian objective of rapamycin complex 1 (mTORC1) bringing about an inhibitory impact on insulin flagging.

Cell Antagonistic Metabolic Result of Supplement Abundance

Under typical conditions, stream of electrons to sub-atomic oxygen, the last acceptor, prompts the siphoning of protons across the internal mitochondrial film, producing a layer potential and proton rationale force that is hence used to drive the blend of ATP from adenosine diphosphate (ADP) and inorganic phosphate. The accessibility of ADP is the main consider deciding the pace of oxidative phosphorylation. Accessibility of ADP is high under states of expanded ATP utilization though electron stream is decreased when ATP necessities are low. Every particle of acetyl CoA created from nonstop oxidation of unsaturated fats, glucose, and amino acids is joined by creation and conveyance of lessening counterparts to the electron transport chain. At the point when ATP utilization is low and ADP accessibility is decreased, this consistent deluge of diminishing reciprocals builds the mitochondrial layer potential and proton slope at last prompting spillage of electrons into the lattice (lessening comparable stock > respiratory demand).Rather than lessening oxygen to water, electrons respond with oxygen to frame superoxide anion followed by fast change to hydrogen peroxide (H2O2) by superoxide dismutase.At low fixations, superoxide creation might be associated with cell signal transduction, yet at high focuses, the revolutionaries make oxidative harm due their high reactivity towards other cell compounds.

Notwithstanding creation along the electron transport chain, H2O2 can likewise be delivered by the pyruvate dehydrogenase complex. Under typical conditions, the glutathione redox buffering network veils most of this creation; be that as it may, under states of a high-fat eating routine, the searching framework becomes oxidized expanding the outflow pace of H2O2 from the chemical complex. Moreover, an expansion in the NADH/NAD+ proportion, as happens with overnutrition and diminished action, can build H2O2 creation by the alpha-ketoglutarate dehydrogenase complex. These extra wellsprings of H2O2 under states of overnutrition make microenvironments helpful for injury.

One more result of the rising NADH/NAD+ratio is an inhibitory impact on a few chemical frameworks in the TCA cycle This impact optionally prompts gathering of acetyl CoA because of easing back transition and diminishing substrate accessibility in the cycle. For instance, utilization of acetyl CoA by citrate synthase diminishes in light of the fact that this compound must initially tie oxaloacetate, which can be restricting because of easing back of the cycle. The catalyst is additionally restrained by succinyl CoA, which is created in expanding sums from digestion of the extended chain amino acids valine and isoleucine, as happens when combinations of energizes are consistently being catabolized. As acetyl CoA collects, it can go about as an acyl contributor and through enzymatic and non-enzymatic systems cause adjustment of proteins like lysine acetylation, succinylation, and palmitoylation. The specific cosmetics of these alterations changes as indicated by the constituents of the eating regimen. As implied, there are buffering instrument recognized which act to limit pernicious impacts of superoxide extremist arrangement and protein adjustments because of acetylation. These incorporate glutathione and thioredoxin-diminishing frameworks, the carnitine framework, and the sirtuin group of NAD+-subordinate deacylases. Regardless of defensive frameworks, supplement over-burden through oxidative pressure and acetylation and protein change compromise the uprightness and pliancy of the fuel switch components prompting a drowsy metabolic reaction to dietary signs.

Metabolic Firmness and Insulin Obstruction

Metabolic firmness is related with insulin obstruction; be that as it may, which one causes the other is as yet unsettled. As per the Randle speculation, expanding the stockpile and oxidation of unsaturated fats creates more acetyl-CoA in the mitochondria and accordingly builds how much citrate accessible for transport into the cytosol. Citrate applies a direct inhibitory impact on phosphofructokinase movement causing collection of glucose 6-phosphate, which thus hinders hexokinase action, bringing about diminished net glucose take-up. Notwithstanding hindrance of glycolysis and glucose oxidation, tissue gathering of lipid and lipid-determined flagging particles, for example, ceramides and diacylglycerol disturb insulin flagging pathways causing diminished movement of glucose carrier type 4 (GLUT4) into the phone layer. gathering is expected to mitochondrial brokenness prompting lacks of oxidative digestion and redirection of unsaturated fats from oxidation and towards creation of poisonous lipid species. As recently referenced, insulin opposition might be a reason for metabolic rigidity and not an outcome.

Insulin responsiveness is likewise impacted by energy expenditure.This relationship can be seen as a continuum where the seriousness of insulin opposition increments as a component of carbon and electron supply comparative with ATP interest across the mitochondria. Expanding supply without an adjustment of interest encroaches upon redox balance deteriorating insulin activity. On the other hand, when expanded ATP request is answerable for expanded β-oxidation and supply of carbon and electrons, metabolic equilibrium is kept up with across the mitochondria and insulin awareness is safeguarded.

Muscle Lipid Content and Insulin Obstruction: The Competitor's Conundrum
In light of the prior conversation, statement of fat in non-fat tissue might possibly be related with insulin opposition and metabolic entanglements of stoutness (lipotoxicity). With regards to stoutness and type 2 diabetes mellitus, intramyocellular triacylglycerol (IMTG) content relates straightforwardly with muscle insulin obstruction and fills in as serious areas of strength for an of diabetes risk. Conversely, the skeletal muscle of prepared perseverance competitors is

notably insulin delicate and has a high oxidative limit, regardless of having raised lipid content. The more noteworthy insulin awareness regardless of a raised IMTG testimony in the perseverance prepared state is alluded to as the competitor's mystery.

Contrasts in muscle fiber type as well as size, subcellular compartmentalization, and practical and underlying contrasts in lipid bead qualities might represent the noticed contrasts between IMTG stockpiling and skeletal muscle insulin responsiveness in the perseverance prepared and insulin safe state.In one review, blended muscle lipid content was considerably more prominent in perseverance competitors when contrasted and stationary sort 2 diabetes patients and their weight matched normoglycemic controls.Only roughly 40% of the more noteworthy blended muscle lipid content was credited to a higher extent of type I muscle strands in the perseverance competitors contrasted and those with type 2 diabetes, though the leftover distinction was made sense of by a fundamentally more prominent IMTG content in the kind I muscle filaments of the prepared competitors. Type 1 filaments are slow-jerk oxidative strands known to contain more all out lipid and a more noteworthy number of mitochondria when contrasted and type 2 quick jerk glycolytic filaments. Lipid collection in type 1 filaments fills in as a promptly accessible wellspring of energy during exercise.

In patients with type 2 diabetes, lipid beads are bigger and are specially put away in the subsarcolemmal district of type II strands, though perseverance prepared subjects store lipid in a larger number of lipid drops that are more modest in size and essentially situated in the intermyofibrillar locale of type I fibers.Increased measures of the covering protein, perilipin 5, act to select and keep up with nearness of the intermyofibrillar drops to mitochondria and safeguard against high-fat eating routine prompted lipotoxicity.Intramyocellular triacylglycerol content reductions during delayed submaximal work out, and comparably to glycogen, intramyocellular lipid content is expanded in the prepared state. Rather than the unique idea of IMTG exhaustion and capacity in the prepared competitor, IMTG stores in the large or potentially type 2 diabetes patient are stale and a sign of a primary lopsidedness between plasma free unsaturated fat accessibility, unsaturated fat (FA) stockpiling, and oxidation. Bigger lipid bead size limits availability to intramyocellular lipases and the subsarcolemmal area might make actual prevention movement of Excess 4 into the cell film adding to insulin opposition. The stale idea of IMTG prompts gathering of fatty substance and FA metabolites, for example, ceramide that further adding to insulin obstruction.

Treatment of Metabolic Rigidity

The key objective in treating metabolic rigidity is to alleviate the decreasing strain and development of receptive oxidation species coming about because of carbon over-burden across the mitochondria. A hypothetical method for achieving this objective is to forestall oxidative digestion of one of three significant fuel sources to bring down carbon import to the mitochondria and ease substrate rivalry. Discontinuous fasting as talked about beneath is the most clinically pertinent method for restricting mitochondrial carbon conveyance. On the other hand, one can endeavor to improve the buffering limit of the different frameworks that effectively moderate mitochondrial reductive pressure. These procedures community on expanding cell reinforcement guard, recovery of glutathione, carnitine-intervened acyl bunch buffering, and sirtuin-intervened protein deacylation.A third and seemingly the best methodology to address the energy irregularity welcomed on by supplement excess is to increment energy interest .This technique guarantees metabolic equilibrium and insulin responsiveness are kept up with in a setting where transition through β-oxidation is expanded.

2: Improving Your Metabolic Flexibility

Further developing metabolic adaptability is without a doubt a gainful objective for by and large wellbeing. Metabolic adaptability alludes to the capacity of our bodies to effectively switch between utilizing different fuel sources, for example, carbs and fats, in view of our energy needs. The following are a couple of tips to assist with working on metabolic adaptability:

1.Balanced Eating regimen: Guarantee you consume an even eating regimen that incorporates a decent blend of starches, proteins, and solid fats. Incorporate different organic products, vegetables, entire grains, lean meats, fish, nuts, and seeds in your eating routine.

2.Proper Hydration: Remaining very much hydrated is significant for keeping up with ideal metabolic capability. Try to hydrate over the course of the day to keep yourself appropriately hydrated.

3.Regular Activity: Standard active work assumes a significant part in working on metabolic adaptability. Take part in a blend of vigorous activities, strength preparing, and extreme cardio exercise (HIIT) to upgrade your body's capacity to use different energy sources proficiently.

4.Intermittent Fasting: Consider integrating irregular fasting into your daily practice. This includes cycling between times of eating and fasting, which can assist with working on the body's usage of put away energy and improve metabolic adaptability.

5.Get Adequate Rest: Focus on getting sufficient quality rest every evening. Deficient rest can upset your digestion and influence your body's capacity to really switch between fuel sources.

6.Manage Pressure: Constant pressure can adversely influence metabolic adaptability. Track down sound ways of overseeing pressure, for example, rehearsing care, taking part in unwinding procedures, or partaking in exercises that you appreciate.

3.Met Flex Recipes:

Met Flex Recipes are an assortment of recipes intended for the Metabolic Adaptability diet. This diet centers around enhancing metabolic adaptability, which is the body's capacity to switch between consuming carbs and fat for fuel proficiently. The recipes are ordinarily adjusted in macronutrients (carbs, proteins, fats) and incorporate various fixings to help in general wellbeing and prosperity. They are frequently custom fitted to explicit dietary requirements and inclinations while as yet advancing metabolic adaptability.

1.Quinoa Veggie Broiled Rice: A solid curve on an exemplary dish, utilizing quinoa rather than rice and stacked with bright vegetables.

2.Lentil and Vegetable Curry: A tasty and protein-pressed curry made with lentils, blended vegetables, and fragrant flavors.

3.Chickpea Serving of mixed greens Wraps: A light and invigorating wrap loaded up with a combination of chickpeas, crunchy vegetables, and a tart dressing.

4.Mushroom and Dark Bean Tacos: A delightful and fulfilling taco filling made with sautéed mushrooms, dark beans, and flavors.

5.Sweet Potato and Dark Bean Burger: A hand crafted veggie burger made with squashed yams, dark beans, and different spices and flavors.

6.Cauliflower Steak: A good and nutritious dish where thick cuts of cauliflower are cooked until brilliant and finished off with a flavorful sauce.

7.Zucchini Noodles with Pesto: A low-carb option in contrast to pasta, made by spiralizing zucchini and throwing it with natively constructed or locally acquired pesto sauce.

8.Veggie Sautéed food: A fast and simple sautéed food dish stacked with a grouping of beautiful vegetables, prepared with soy sauce or teriyaki sauce.

9.Spinach and Feta Stuffed Peppers: Simmered chime peppers loaded down with a combination of sautéed spinach, feta cheddar, and breadcrumbs.

10.Lentil Shepherd's Pie: A vegan variant of the exemplary dish, made with lentils, vegetables, and finished off with pureed potatoes.

4.Exercises

Meta-flex practices allude to a sort of unique extending that objectives various muscle gatherings and upgrades adaptability. These activities center around expanding the scope of movement and further developing portability in different pieces of the body. Meta-flex practices include constant development, frequently integrating components of extending, versatility, and strength-building exercises.

The vital advantages of meta-flex practices include:

1.Improved adaptability: Meta-flex practices help to extend and extend muscles, ligaments, and tendons, which can work on your general adaptability and scope of movement.

2.Increased versatility: By focusing on various muscle gatherings and joints at the same time, meta-flex activities can improve your joint portability and make regular developments simpler.

3.Injury avoidance: Normal act of meta-flex activities can assist with forestalling wounds by expanding joint strength and adaptability, decreasing muscle lopsided characteristics, and further developing body mindfulness.

4.Enhanced execution: Meta-flex practices are ordinarily involved by competitors and wellness aficionados to further develop execution in sports and other proactive tasks. They can assist with improving muscle actuation, power, and coordination.

A few instances of meta-flex practices include:

1.Walking jumps with a wind: Perform strolling rushes while turning your middle to the side of the lead leg, extending the hip flexors, and initiating the center muscles.

2.Inchworms: Begin in a standing position, twist forward, and walk your hands out until you are in a high board position. Then, at that point, walk your feet towards your hands, getting back to the beginning position. This exercise focuses on the hamstrings, center, and chest area.

3.Spiderman slithers: Expect a push-up position and bring your right foot up to the beyond your right hand while keeping a low position. Rehash on the opposite side, rotating this way and that. This exercise advances hip portability, extends the crotch, and connects with the chest area and center.

Make sure to heat up prior to performing meta-flex activities and begin with lower power developments on the off chance that you're a novice. It's likewise fundamental to keep up with legitimate structure and pay attention to your body to abstain from overextending or overexertion. On the off chance that you have any prior ailments or concerns, talk with a medical care proficient prior to beginning another work-out daily schedule.

5.Snacks

Met Flex snacks are a sort of high-protein bites that are intended to help a functioning and sound way of life. These bites are frequently well known among wellness fans or those searching for a helpful method for expanding their protein consumption.

Met Flex snacks are commonly made with excellent fixings like whey protein, nuts, seeds, and other healthy fixings. They are known for being low in starches and sugar while being wealthy in protein, which makes them an extraordinary choice for those watching their macros or following a high-protein diet.

These bites are accessible in different structures, including protein bars, protein treats, protein chips, and protein shakes. They arrive in many flavors to suit various inclinations. Met Flex bites can be consumed as a fast and helpful in a hurry nibble, pre-or post-exercise fuel, or as a better option in contrast to customary tidbits.

It's quite important that while Met Flex bites can be a helpful expansion to a solid eating routine, they shouldn't supplant entire food sources in your eating routine. It is generally essential to keep a decent and differed diet to guarantee you get every one of the important supplements your body needs.

Conclusion

The Met Flex dietary propensities center around augmenting calorie consume and improving fuel for the body. By following these propensities, people can accomplish their weight and wellness objectives successfully. The vital standards of the Met Flex approach incorporate expanding metabolic adaptability, consolidating supplement thick food varieties, and rehearsing key fasting or time-limited eating. These propensities help in consuming more calories as well as furnish the body with excellent fuel to help in general wellbeing and execution. It is encouraged to talk with a medical services proficient or an enlisted dietitian prior to rolling out any huge improvements to your dietary propensities.